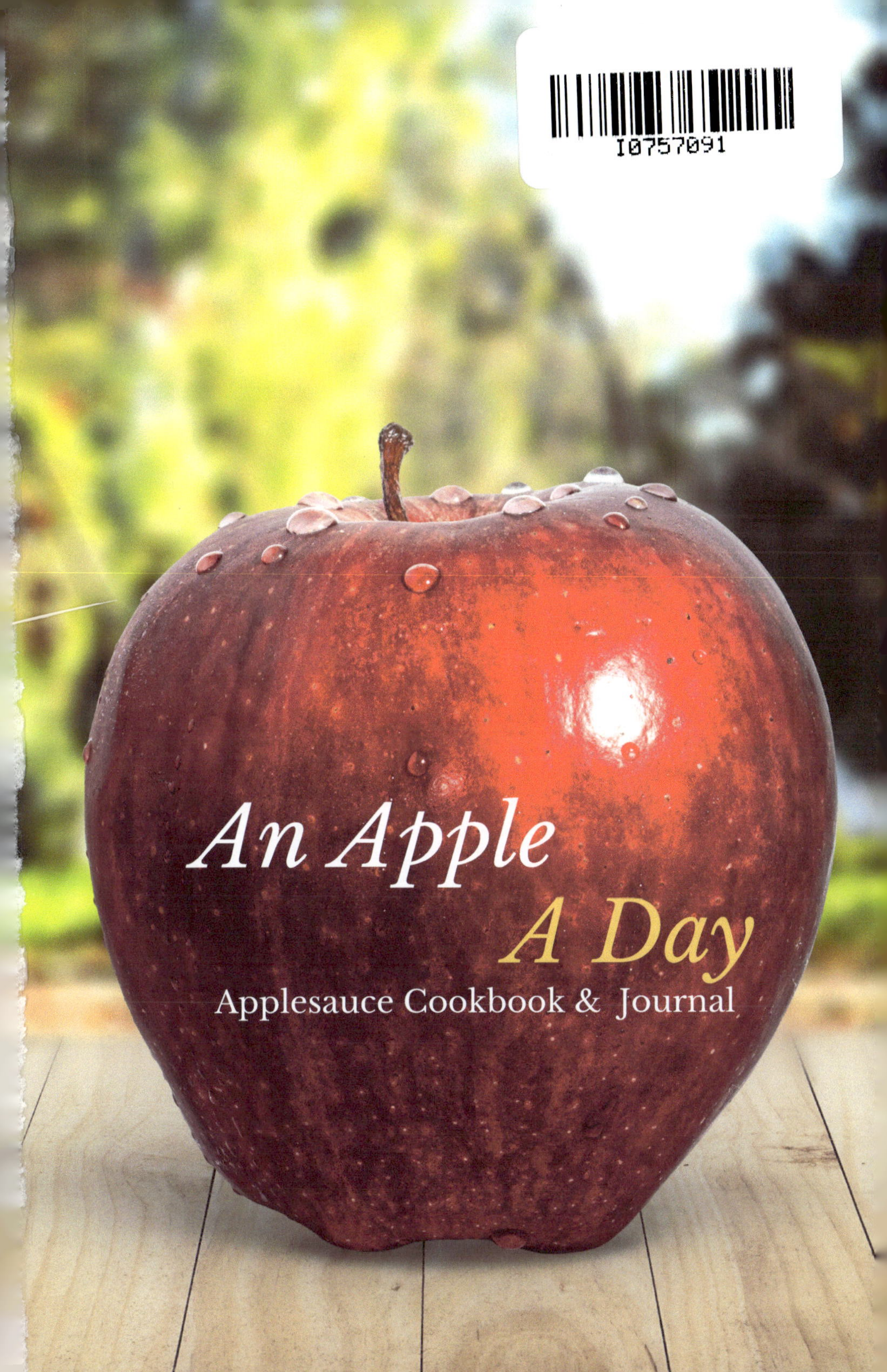

I0757091
An Apple
A Day
Applesauce Cookbook & Journal

This book is a compilation of some of my most favorite applesauce recipes using my very own brand, MRS. MARCY'S HOMEMADES. From gourmet desserts, nutritious snacks, cooking substitutes and more, APPLESAUCE is the unsung hero of your pantry.

During the height of the COVID 19 global pandemic, one thing became obvious – we all must be healthy in order to live longer. We took for granted that we would live forever – now is the season of "being woke". The earth has all we need, its time to take back control of our health.

APPLESAUCE IT IS!!

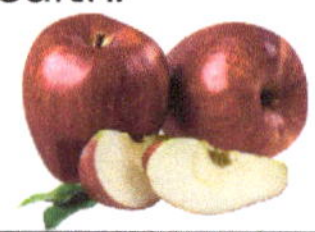

Deepest thanks to my family. My husband Robert – he likes to claim an apple hit him on the head and he came up with the idea. (laugh) I'll let him hold onto that notion. He has been my rock! Through the countless tears, back and shoulder pain, numerous NOs, he continued to encourage me. Even when I threaten to fire him, he keeps coming back.

My mother – Chief Apple Peeler and fruit washer. She's going to fuss, but at 81 yrs. old, she drives 20 minutes to come help me every time I am making applesauce, cider or cold pressed juices. The time we spend together is priceless and I do not take it for granted.

My daughters Maya and Jazmine. Maya is my conscience. She keeps me straight and healthy. When she comes into the shop to organize, I just step back and let her do what she does best – keep me in order. Jazmine is my voice of reason. Whenever I share an idea, thought or emotion, she is there to put it into perspective. I know she has my back and is always there as an extra support.

I would be remised if I did not mention my Assistant Tai. She was my 1st employee and has been there since Day 1. Loyalty is not something you come by often, however I can say her loyalty, respect and excitement for the applesauce is unmatched.

TABLE OF CONTENTS

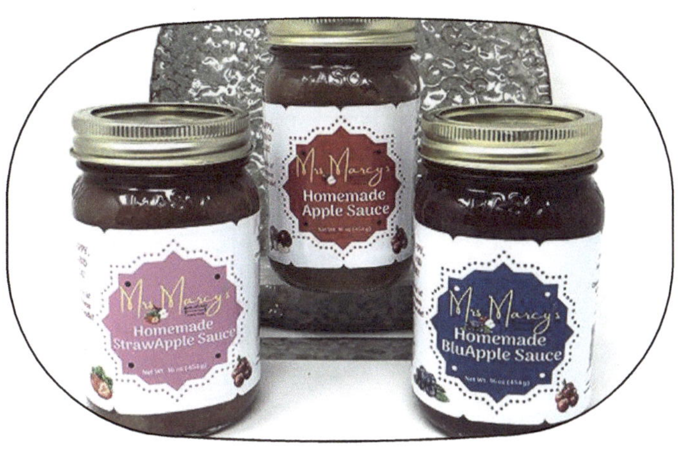

Mrs. Marcy's Homemades, LLC
9550 Midlothian Tnpk., Suite 118
Richmond, VA 23235

www.mrsmarcyshomemades.com | mrsmarcyshomemades@gmail.com

MRS. MARCY'S HOMEMADES

WHAT STARTED AS A QUARANTINE HOBBY FOR MARCY THORNHILL HAS TURNED INTO A GROWING BUSINESS!

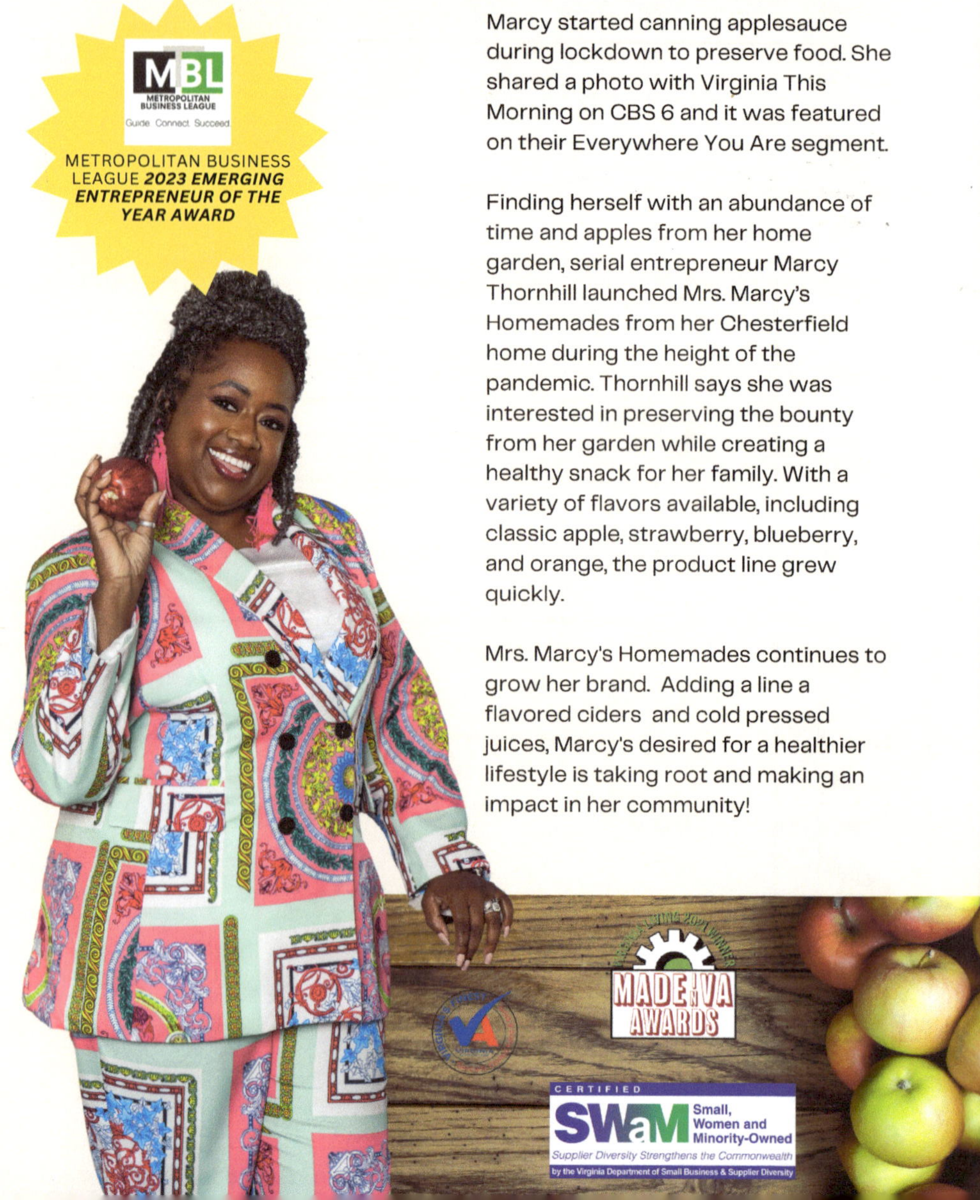

Marcy started canning applesauce during lockdown to preserve food. She shared a photo with Virginia This Morning on CBS 6 and it was featured on their Everywhere You Are segment.

Finding herself with an abundance of time and apples from her home garden, serial entrepreneur Marcy Thornhill launched Mrs. Marcy's Homemades from her Chesterfield home during the height of the pandemic. Thornhill says she was interested in preserving the bounty from her garden while creating a healthy snack for her family. With a variety of flavors available, including classic apple, strawberry, blueberry, and orange, the product line grew quickly.

Mrs. Marcy's Homemades continues to grow her brand. Adding a line a flavored ciders and cold pressed juices, Marcy's desired for a healthier lifestyle is taking root and making an impact in her community!

HEALTH BENEFITS OF
Applesauce

Applesauce is a healthy and delicious snack that provides several health benefits. It is rich in fiber, which promotes digestive health and helps you feel full. Additionally, it contains a variety of vitamins and minerals, such as vitamin C and potassium, that can strengthen your immune system and support heart health. Applesauce is also a great option for those watching their calorie intake, as it is low in calories and fat. Just be sure to choose our vegan varieties to avoid added sugars. Incorporating applesauce into your diet can be a simple way to improve your overall health and wellbeing.

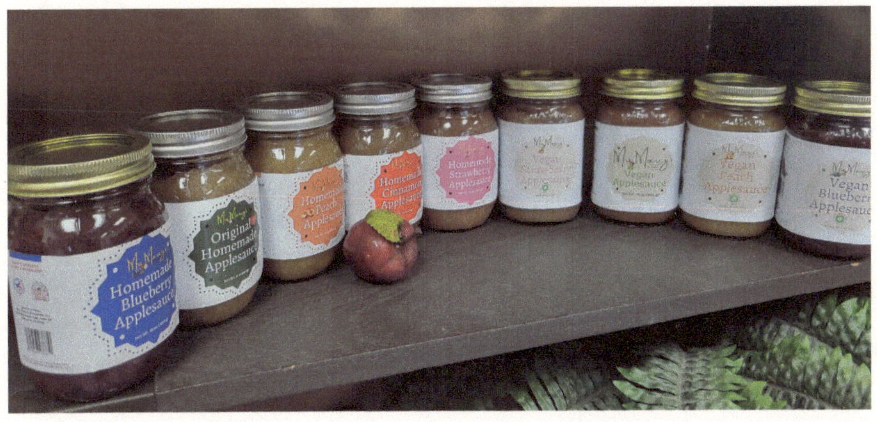

5 Minute Gratitude Journal

__ / __ / ___

S M T W TH F S

Breath before writing

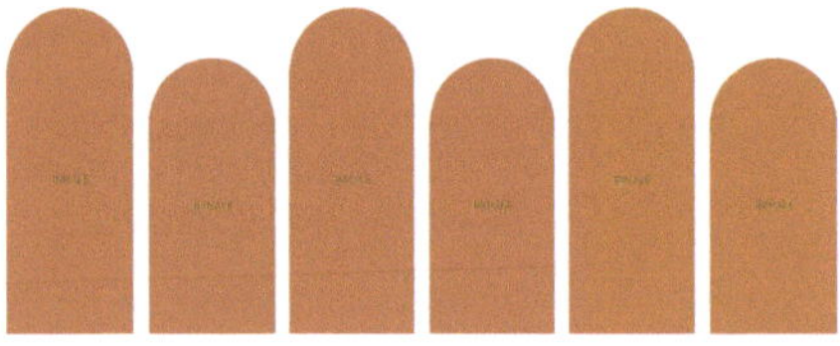

3 best thing about today

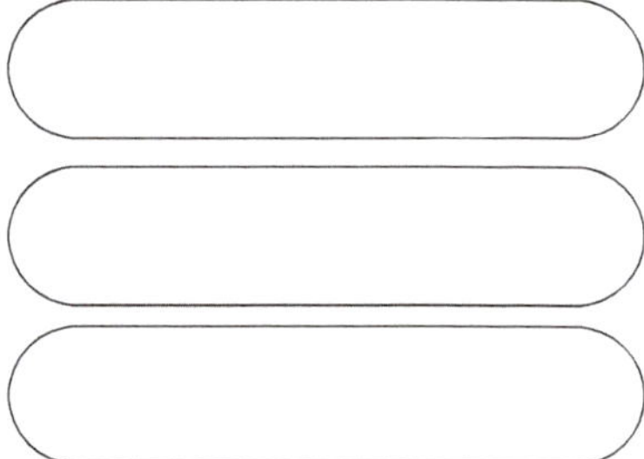

Things you're grateful today

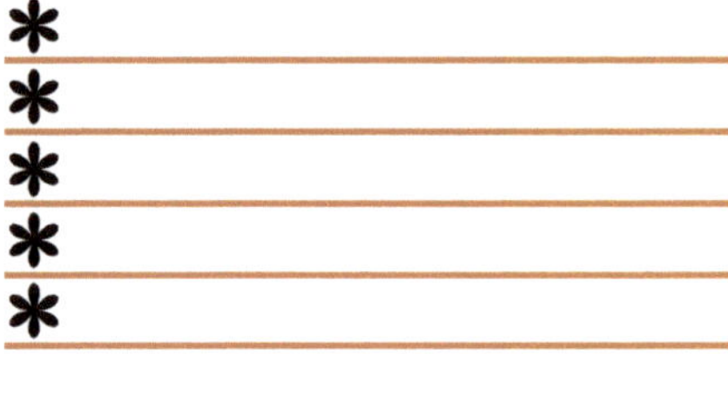

Today's Highlight

Describe today in a drawing

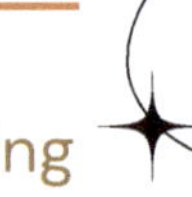

Things that you learned

Today's Affirmation

WEEKLY PLANNER

MONDAY

TUESDAY

WEDNESDAY

THURSDAY

FRIDAY

SATURDAY

TO DO LIST

SUNDAY

NOTES

KEEP GOING!

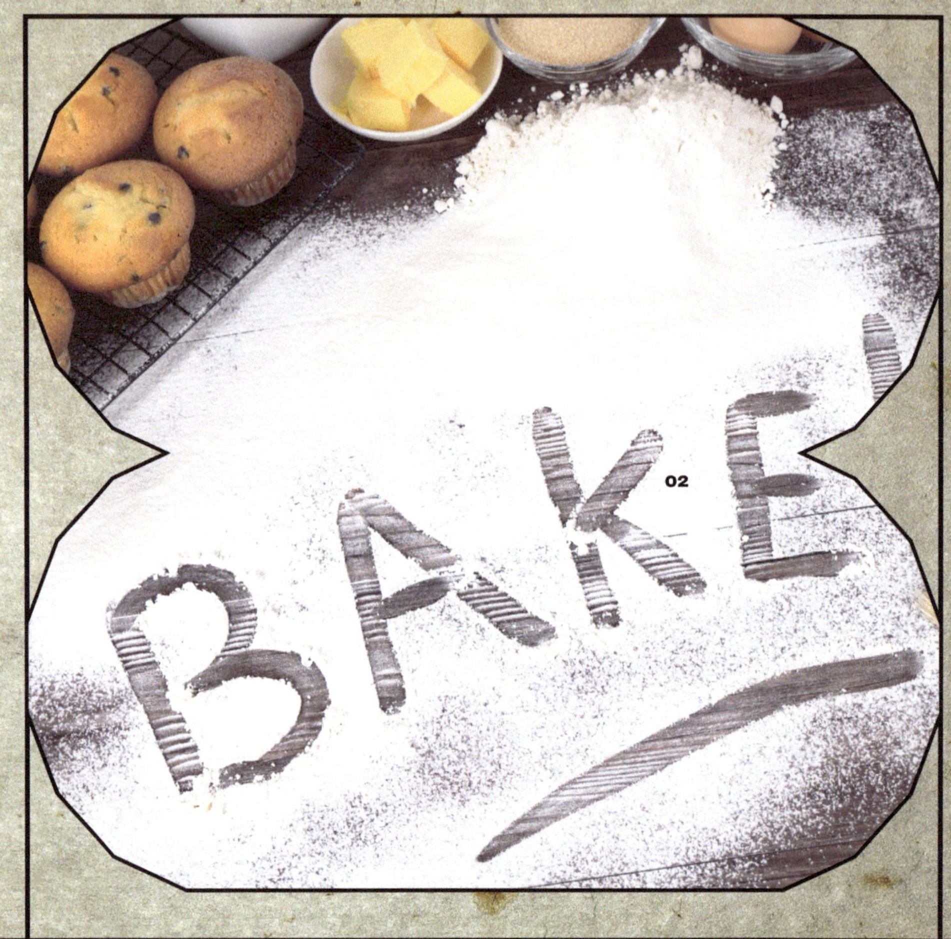

TRY SOME TASTY RECIPES WITH APPLESAUCE. CAKES, COOKIES, MUFFINS, AND MORE ARE ALL BETTER WITH MRS. MARCY'S HOMEMADE APPLESAUCE.

APPLESAUCE Cookies

- 2 cups of all-purpose flour
- 1 teaspoon baking soda
- 1 teaspoon baking powder
- 1/2 teaspoon salt
- 1 teaspoon ground cinnamon
- 1/4 teaspoon ground nutmeg
- 1/2 cup (1 stick) unsalted butter, softened.
- 3/4 cup packed light brown sugar.
- 1/4 cup granulated sugar
- 2 large eggs
- 1 teaspoon pure vanilla extract
- 1 cup applesauce
- 1 cup raisins
- 1/2 cup chopped walnuts

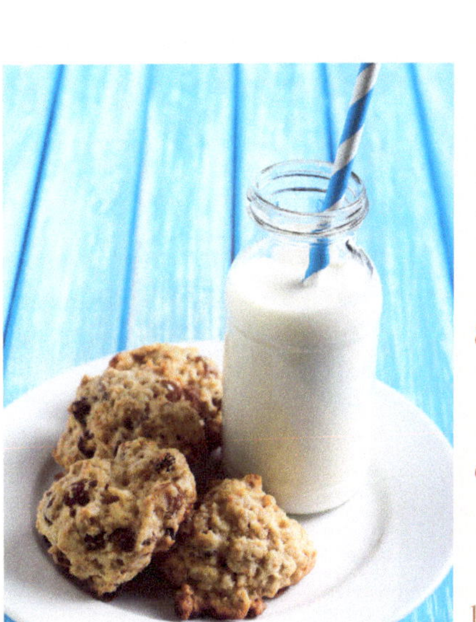

1. Preheat oven to 350°F.

2. Line two baking sheets with parchment paper.

3. In a medium bowl, whisk together the flour, baking soda, baking powder, salt, cinnamon, and nutmeg. Set aside.

4. In the bowl of a stand mixer fitted with the paddle attachment, beat the butter and sugars on medium speed until light and fluffy, about 3 minutes.

5. Add the eggs, one at a time, beating until combined. Beat in the vanilla extract.

6. Reduce the speed to low and add the flour mixture. Beat until just combined.

7. Add the applesauce, raisins, and walnuts, and beat until combined.

8. Drop the dough by the tablespoonful onto the prepared baking sheets, spacing them about 2 inches apart.

9. Bake for 10-12 minutes, until the edges are lightly golden and the centers are just set.

10. Let cool on the baking sheets for 5 minutes before transferring to a wire rack to cool completely. Enjoy!

APPLESAUCE PANCAKES

Ingredients

- 1 cup all-purpose flour
- 1 teaspoon cinnamon
- ½ teaspoon allspice (optional)
- 1 tablespoon baking powder
- 2 tablespoons light brown sugar (or granulated sugar)
- ½ teaspoon <u>kosher salt</u>
- 1 large egg (or <u>flax egg</u> for vegan)
- 1 tablespoon <u>neutral oil</u>
- ¾ cup applesauce
- 2/3 cup milk of choice (2% or non-dairy milk)

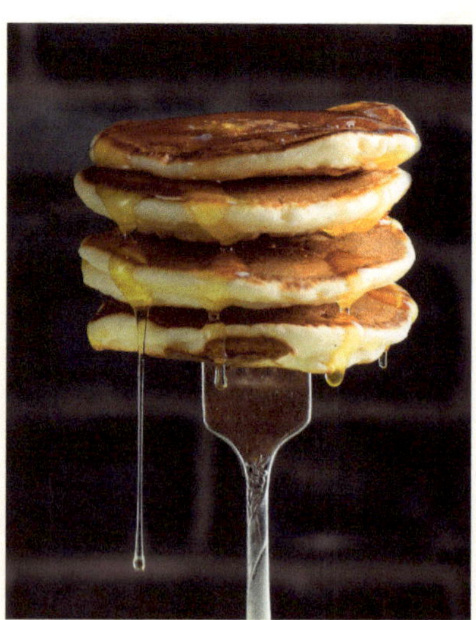

Directions

1. In a medium bowl, whisk together the all purpose flour, cinnamon, allspice (if using), baking powder, sugar, and kosher salt.

2. In another bowl, whisk together the egg, oil, applesauce, and milk.

3. Stir the wet ingredients into the dry ingredients until a smooth, thick batter forms. Lightly grease a skillet with butter and wipe off extra grease with a paper towel. Heat the skillet over low heat. Pour the batter into small circles (a little less than ¼ cup each). Cook the pancakes until the bubbles pop on the top and the bottoms are golden: low and slow is the key! Then flip them and cook until golden on the other side.

If necessary, add a tiny splash of milk to the batter. Repeat with the remaining batter, adjusting the heat as necessary (the skillet can get very hot on the second batch). Place the cooked pancakes under an inverted bowl to keep them warm. Serve immediately with maple syrup.

- **Low and slow is key!** Set the heat on low, or only as high as medium low. Cook them slowly, and they'll come out perfectly cooked on the inside and golden brown on the outside. Don't worry if it feels like it's taking a long time: the extra minute or two is worth it!
- **When to flip? When bubbles form and pop.** Wait until bubbles form on the surface and start to pop. Trust us: this trick works every time!

APPLESAUCE MUFFINS

*"Muffins" backwards describes what you
do when you take them out of the oven*

Ingredients

- 1 and 1/2 cups all-purpose flour
- 1/2 cup sugar
- 1 teaspoon baking powder
- 1/2 teaspoon baking soda
- 1/4 teaspoon salt
- 1/2 teaspoon cinnamon
- 1/2 cup unsweetened applesauce
- 1/4 cup vegetable oil
- 1/4 cup milk
- 1 egg

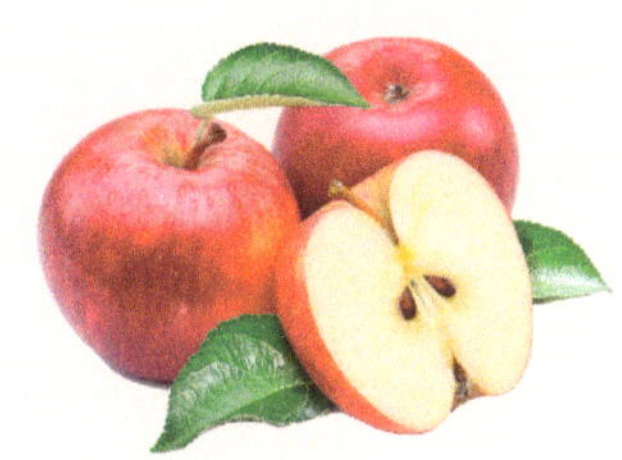

Directions

1. Preheat your oven to 375°F (190°C) and line a muffin tin with paper liners.

2. In a large mixing bowl, whisk together the flour, sugar, baking powder, baking soda, salt, and cinnamon.

3. In a separate bowl, whisk together the applesauce, vegetable oil, milk, and egg until well combined.

4. Pour the wet ingredients into the dry ingredients and stir until just combined. Divide the batter evenly among the muffin cups (about 2/3 full).

5. Bake for 18-20 minutes or until a toothpick inserted into the center of a muffin comes out clean.

6. Allow the muffins to cool in the pan for a few minutes before transferring them to a wire rack to cool completely. Enjoy!

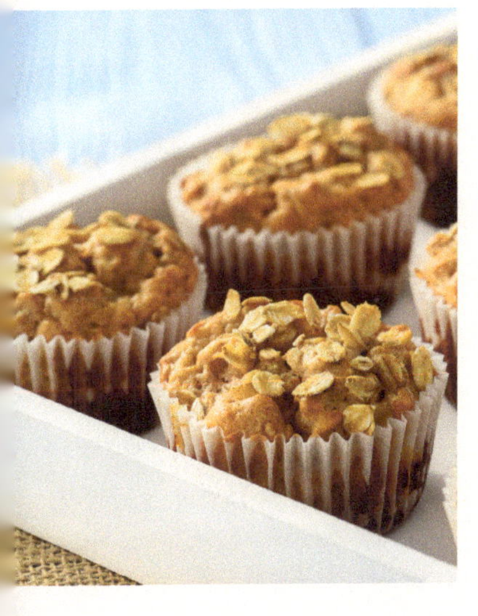

WEEKLY PLANNER

MONDAY

TUESDAY

WEDNESDAY

THURSDAY

FRIDAY

SATURDAY

TO DO LIST

SUNDAY

NOTES

KEEP GOING!

APPLESAUCE CAKE

w/ Box Cake Mix

Applesauce cake is a delicious dessert that is easy to make.

The main ingredient, applesauce, gives the cake a moist texture and a subtle apple flavor.

Ingredients

To make the cake, you will need:

- Mrs. Marcy's Homemades Applesauce
- 18 ¼ ounces sizes Yellow Cake Mix
- 3 Eggs
- 16 ounces sizes

Directions

1. Mix the dry ingredients together, then add the wet ingredients.

2. Pour the batter into a greased cake pan and bake in the oven for about 30–35 minutes.

3. Once the cake is done, let it cool before serving. You can also add frosting or a dusting of powdered sugar for extra sweetness.

Enjoy your homemade applesauce cake!

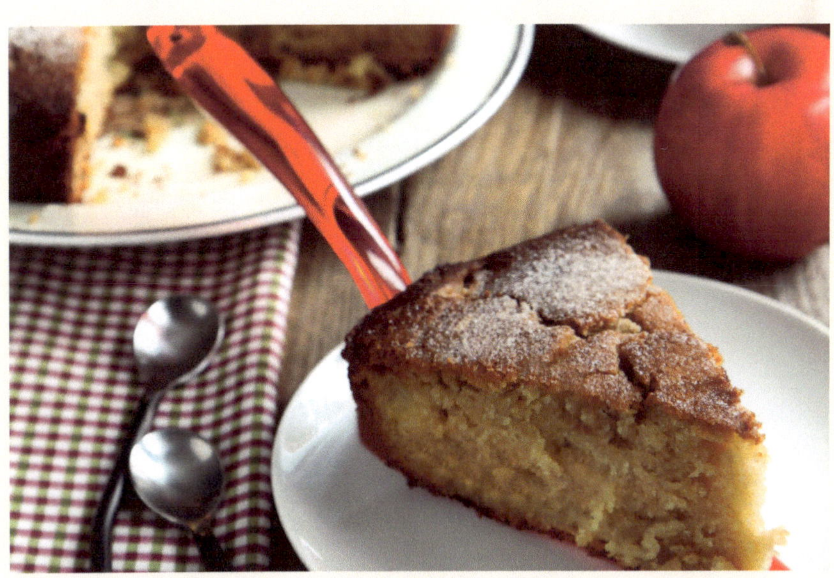

APPLESAUCE STUFFING

Stuffing tastes 10 times better with my favorite secret ingredient: applesauce. This is where sweet and savory live happily ever after!

Ingredients

- 1 loaf of bread, cut into small pieces
- 1 cup of applesauce
- 1/2 cup of chicken broth
- 1/4 cup of butter
- 1 onion, chopped
- 2 stalks of celery, chopped
- 2 tablespoons of fresh parsley, chopped
- Salt and pepper to taste

Directions

1 Preheat the oven to 350°F.

2 Spread the bread pieces out on a baking sheet and bake for 10-15 minutes until they are lightly toasted.

3 In a large skillet, melt the butter over medium-high heat.

4 Add the onion and celery and cook until they are softened, about 5-7 minutes.

5 Add the toasted bread pieces, applesauce, chicken broth, parsley, salt, and pepper to the skillet.

6 Stir until everything is well combined and the bread is coated with the liquid.

7 Pour the mixture into a greased baking dish and bake for 30-35 minutes, until the stuffing is golden brown on top.
Serve hot and enjoy!

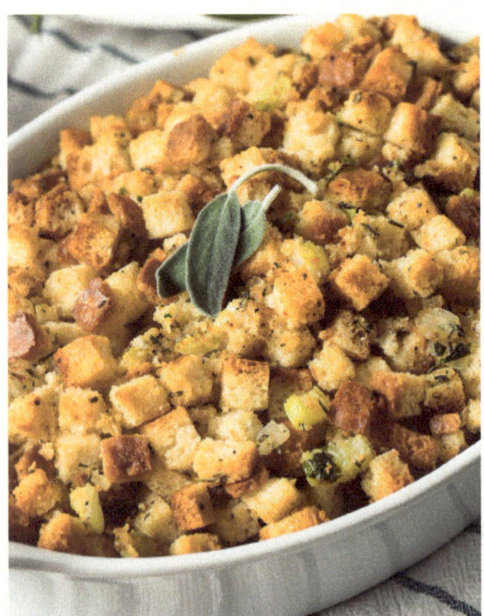

WEEKLY PLANNER

MONDAY

TUESDAY

WEDNESDAY

THURSDAY

FRIDAY

SATURDAY

TO DO LIST

SUNDAY

NOTES

KEEP GOING!

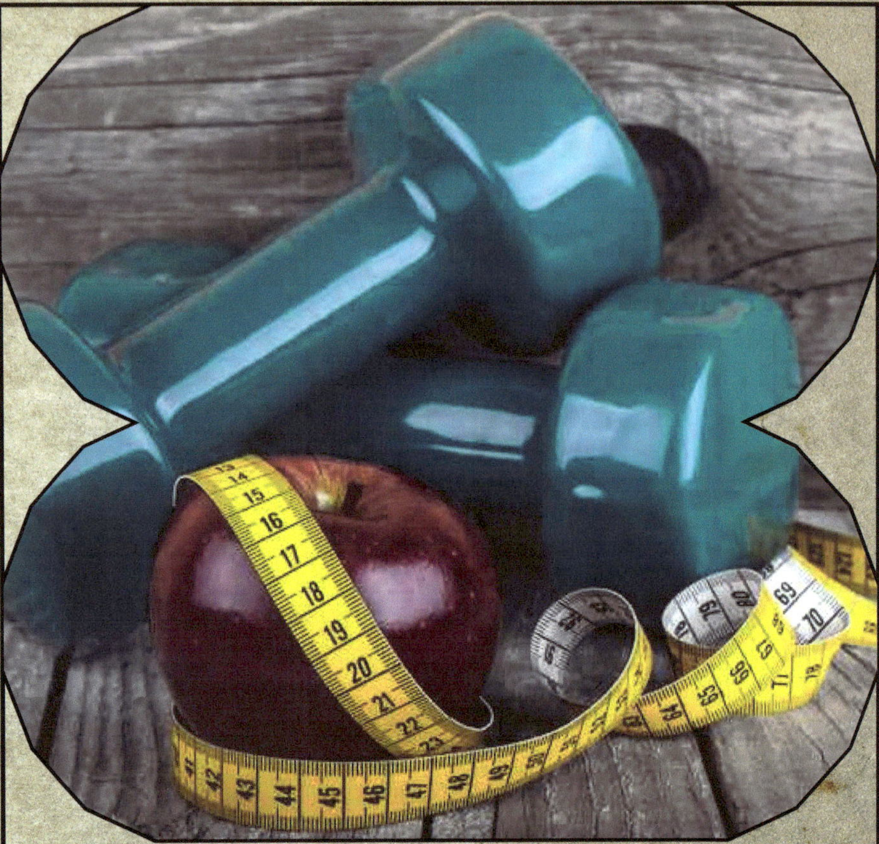

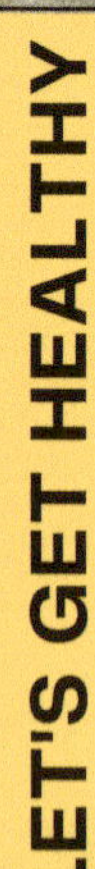

APPLESAUCE: A HEALTHY SNACK CHOICE

5 Minute Gratitude Journal

__/__/___

S M T W TH F S

Breath before writing

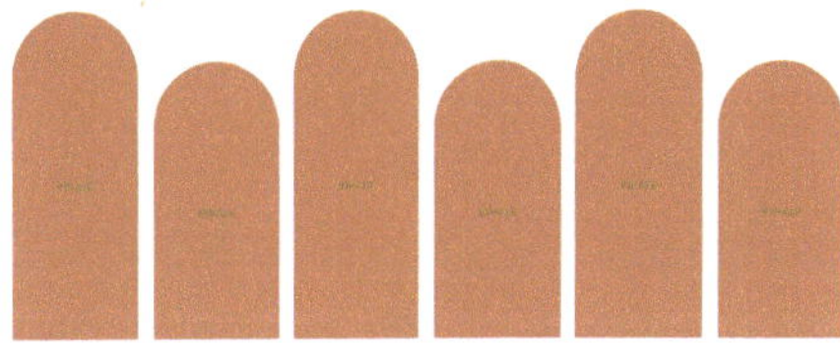

3 best thing about today

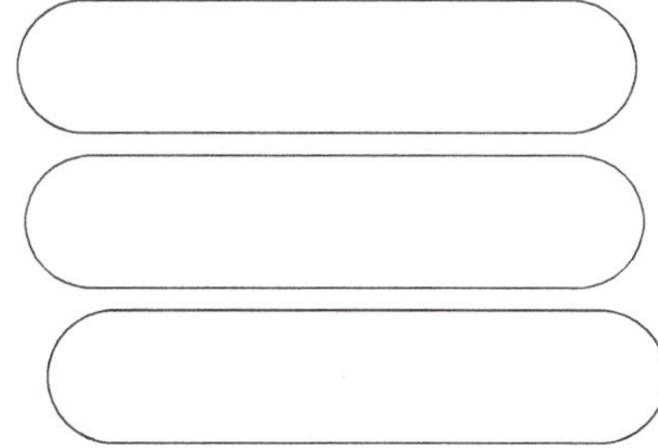

Things you're grateful today

*
*
*
*
*

Describe today in a drawing

Today's Highlight

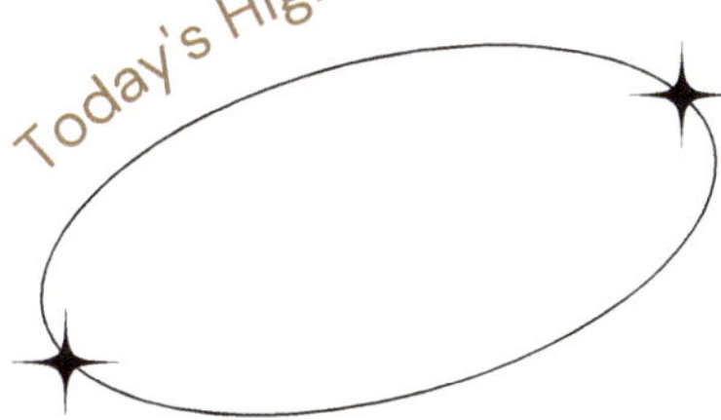

Things that you learned

Today's Affirmation

Today I'm grateful for...

APPLESAUCE ENERGY BAR

The applesauce energy bar is a nutritious snack that can provide a quick boost of energy. It is typically made with ingredients such as oats, nuts, seeds, and of course, applesauce. This type of energy bar is a popular choice among athletes and fitness enthusiasts as it can help fuel their workouts. Additionally, it can also be a convenient and healthy snack option for people on-the-go or those looking to maintain a balanced diet. Overall, the applesauce energy bar is a delicious and nutritious snack that can provide a variety of health benefits.

Ingredients

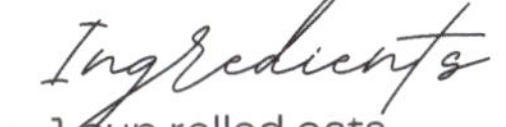

- 1 cup rolled oats
- 1/2 cup unsweetened applesauce
- 1/4 cup honey
- 1/4 cup almond butter
- 1/4 cup chopped almonds
- 1/4 cup dried cranberries
- 1/4 cup chocolate chips
- 1 tsp cinnamon

Directions

1. Preheat the oven to 350°F (180°C) and line a baking pan with parchment paper.

2. In a large bowl, mix together the oats, applesauce, honey, and almond butter until well combined.

3. Stir in the chopped almonds, dried cranberries, chocolate chips, and cinnamon.

4. Pour the mixture into the prepared baking pan and press it evenly into the pan.

5. Bake for 20-25 minutes, or until the edges are lightly golden brown. Let the bars cool completely in the pan before cutting into squares.

6. Store the bars in an airtight container for up to a week. Enjoy as a healthy snack on-the-go!

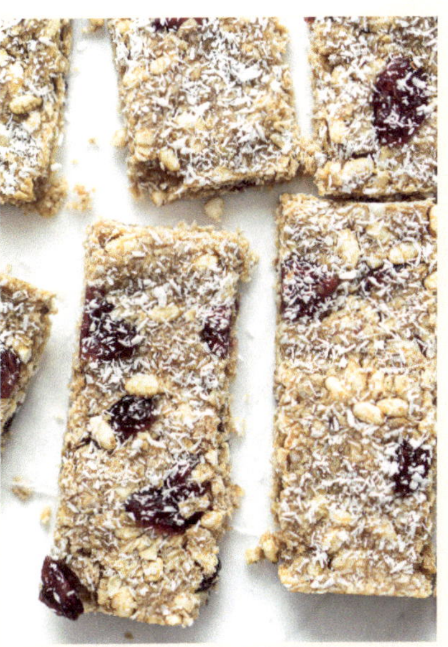

SMOOTHIE

Ingredients

1 cup white sugar
½ cup butter
1 cup chilled applesauce
2 cups all-purpose flour
1 teaspoon baking soda
1 teaspoon ground cinnamon
¼ teaspoon ground cloves
½ cup chopped walnuts
½ cup raisins

This sweet and creamy applesauce smoothie is so delicious and easy to make!

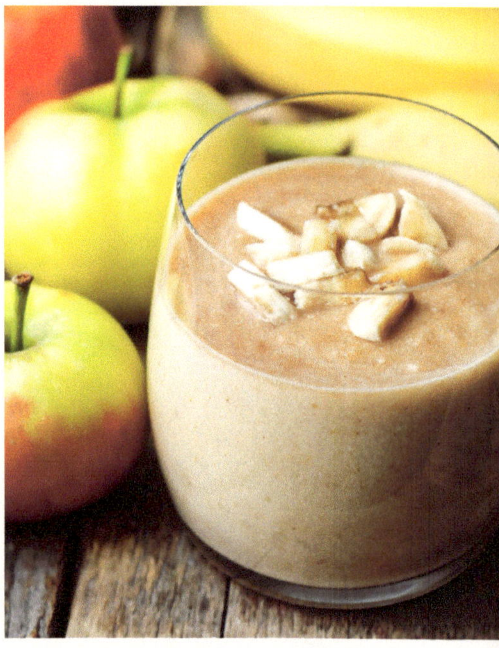

Directions

1. Applesauce smoothie is a delicious and healthy beverage that can be easily made at home.

2. To make this smoothie, simply blend applesauce, yogurt, milk, and honey until smooth. You can also add a dash of cinnamon for extra flavor.

3. This smoothie is a great way to get your daily dose of fruit and protein and makes for a perfect breakfast or snack.

4. Give it a try and enjoy the refreshing taste of this homemade applesauce smoothie!

Today I'm grateful for...

APPLESAUCE BAKED BEANS

Healthier than the instant stuff, but with the same level of convenience.

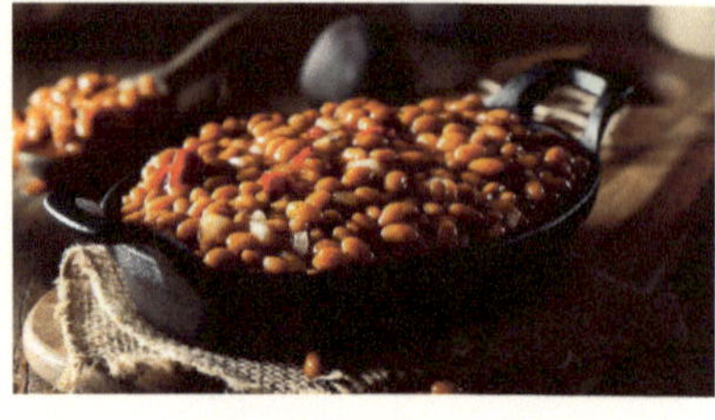

Ingredients

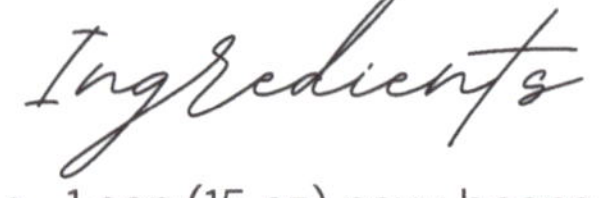

- 1 can (15 oz) navy beans, drained and rinsed
- 1 can (15 oz) red kidney beans, drained and rinsed
- 1 can (15 oz) black beans, drained and rinsed
- 1/2 cup unsweetened applesauce
- 1/2 cup ketchup
- 1/4 cup brown sugar
- 1 tablespoon Worcestershire sauce
- 1 teaspoon mustard powder
- 1/2 teaspoon garlic powder
- Salt and black pepper to taste

1. Preheat the oven to 350°F.

2. In a bowl, mix together the applesauce, ketchup, brown sugar, Worcestershire sauce, mustard powder, garlic powder, salt, and black pepper.

3. Add the beans to the bowl and stir until well combined.

4. Transfer the mixture to a 9x13 inch baking dish and smooth out the top.

5. Bake for 45-50 minutes, or until the beans are hot and bubbly.

6. Let cool for a few minutes before serving.

7. Enjoy your delicious and easy-to-make applesauce baked beans!

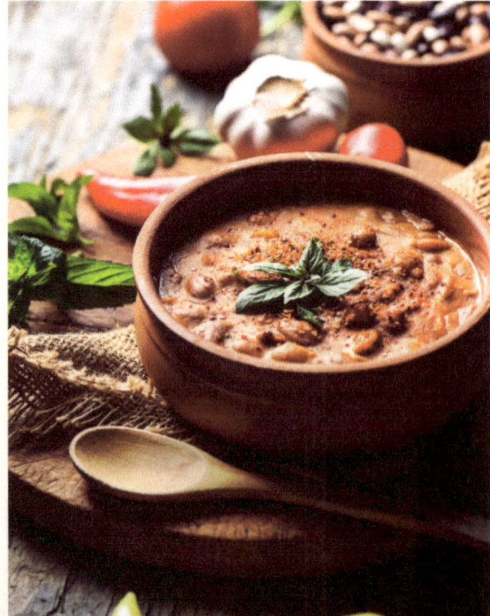

HEALTH BENEFITS OF
Strawberries

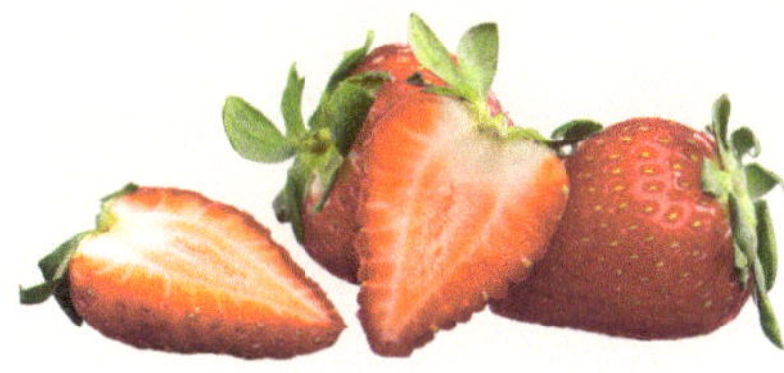

Strawberries are a great source of nutrients and have numerous health benefits.
They are low in calories, high in fiber, and packed with vitamins and minerals.
Eating strawberries can help improve heart health by reducing inflammation and improving blood pressure levels.

They also contain antioxidants that help protect against cancer and other chronic diseases.

Additionally, strawberries have been shown to improve brain function and memory, as well as promote healthy skin and hair. Incorporating strawberries into your diet can be a delicious and nutritious way to improve your overall health.

1Amazing Health Benefits of Strawberries
1. Strawberries Enhance Cognitive Function
2. Strawberries Benefit Diabetics
3. Strawberries Protect the Heart
4. Strawberries Reduce Hypertension
5. Strawberry Can Help Prevent Allergies and Asthma
6. Strawberry Improve Eyesight
7. Strawberry Strengthen The Immune System

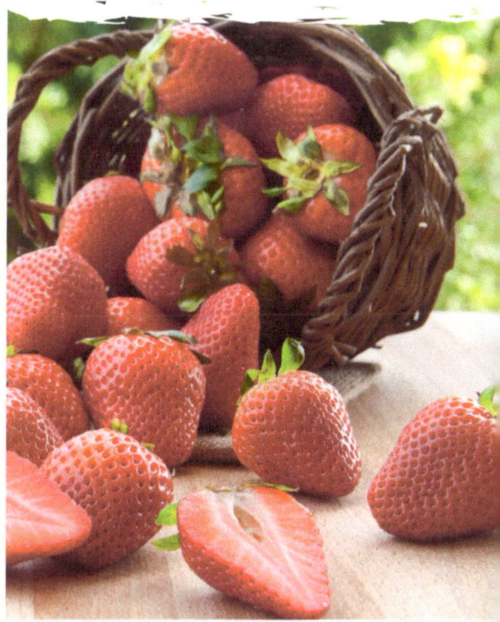

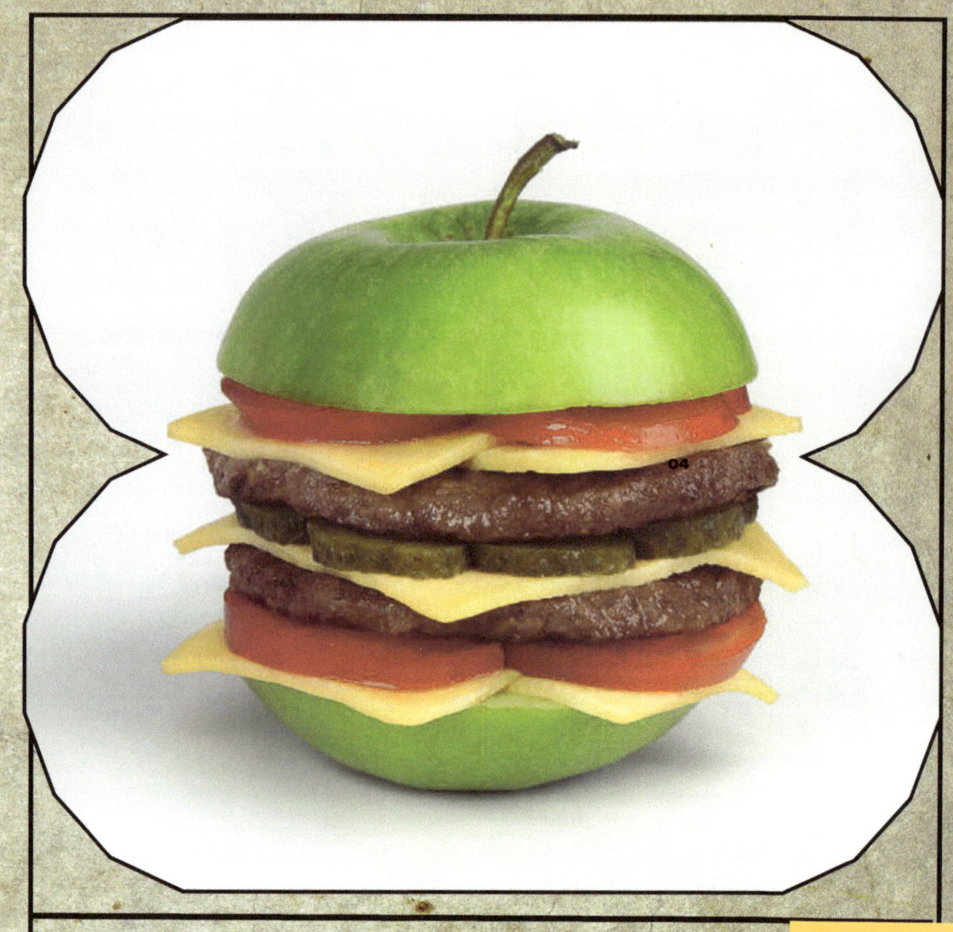

"BURGERS: THE PERFECT BALANCE OF SIMPLICITY AND SATISFACTION."

20

HOW TO USE APPLESAUCE IN
BURGERS

Applesauce can be used in burgers as a healthy and flavorful alternative to traditional condiments. To incorporate it into your burger recipe, simply mix a few tablespoons of unsweetened applesauce into the ground beef before forming the patties. This will add moisture and sweetness to the burgers without adding extra fat or sugar. You can also use applesauce as a topping by spreading it onto the bun or mixing it with other toppings like mustard or mayonnaise.

Ingredients

- 1 lb ground beef
- 1/4 cup applesauce
- 1/4 cup breadcrumbs
- 1/4 cup chopped onion
- 1/4 cup chopped parsley
- 1 egg
- Salt and pepper
- Burger buns
- Toppings of your choice

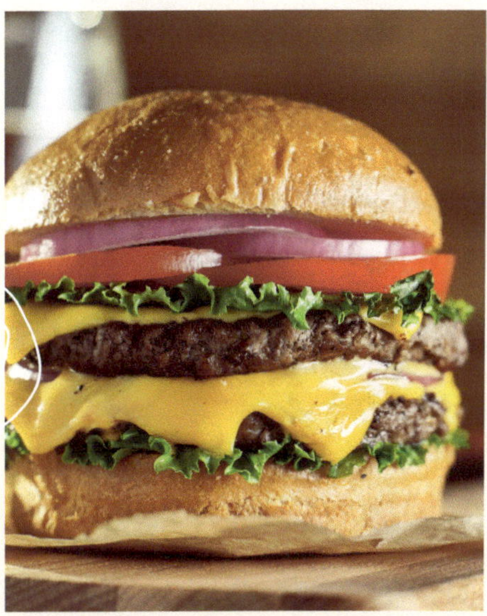

We go together like burger and applesauce

1. In a large bowl, mix together ground beef, applesauce, breadcrumbs, onion, parsley, egg, salt, and pepper.

2. Divide the mixture into 4 equal portions and shape into patties.

3. Heat a grill or a grill pan over medium-high heat.

4. Grill the burgers for about 5-7 minutes on each side, or until they are cooked to your liking.

5. Toast the burger buns and assemble the burgers with your favorite toppings.

Enjoy your delicious applesauce burger!

HOW TO USE APPLESAUCE TO MARINATE CHICKEN

1 cup of applesauce
1/4 cup of soy sauce
1/4 cup of honey
1 tablespoon of Dijon mustard
2 cloves of minced garlic.

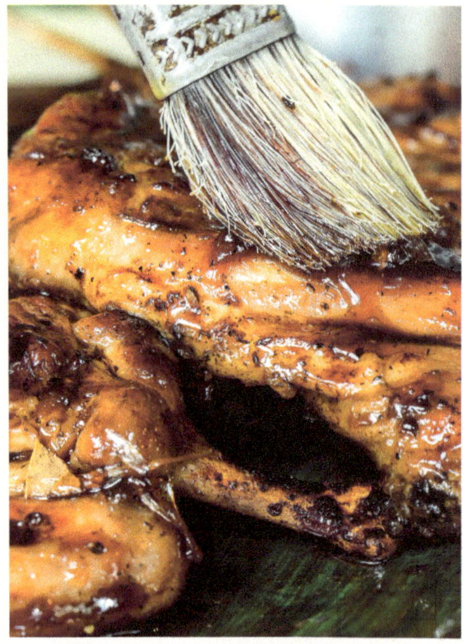

1 In a bowl, mix 1 cup of applesauce, 1/4 cup of soy sauce, 1/4 cup of honey, 1 tablespoon of Dijon mustard, and 2 cloves of minced garlic.

2 Place chicken in a large resealable bag and pour the marinade over it, making sure the chicken is evenly coated.

3 Refrigerate for at least 2 hours, or overnight for best results.

4 When ready to cook, preheat grill to medium–high heat and cook chicken for 6-8 minutes on each side, or until fully cooked.

5 To use applesauce as a marinade for chicken, mix the applesauce with other flavorings such as garlic, soy sauce, honey, or vinegar.

6 Place the chicken in a resealable plastic bag and pour the marinade over it, making sure all the chicken pieces are coated.

7 Close the bag tightly and refrigerate for at least 30 minutes, or up to 24 hours for more flavor.

8 When you're ready to cook the chicken, discard the marinade and grill, bake, or sauté the chicken as desired.

The applesauce marinade will add a sweet and tangy flavor to the chicken.

Enjoy your delicious and flavorful applesauce chicken!

HEALTH BENEFITS OF
Blueberries

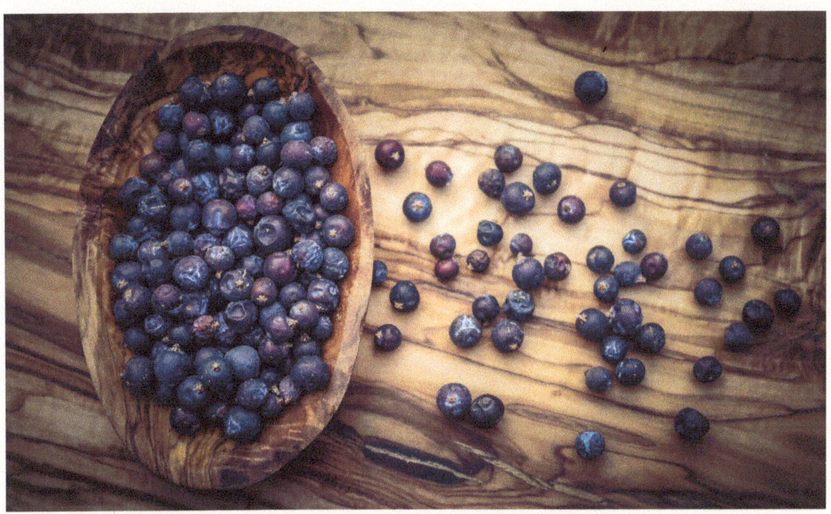

Blueberries are a superfood that offer numerous health benefits. They are packed with antioxidants that can help reduce inflammation and improve heart health. Blueberries are also rich in vitamins C and K, and dietary fiber, which can aid in digestion and promote healthy skin. Additionally, blueberries have been shown to improve cognitive function and protect against age-related cognitive decline. Incorporating blueberries into your diet is an easy way to reap these health benefits.

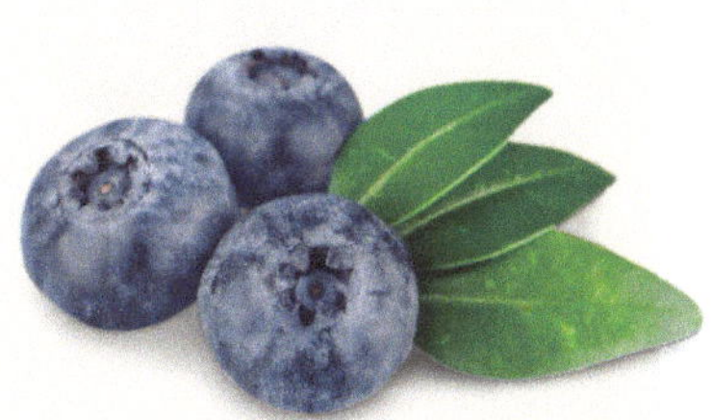

According to a 2004 study, a cup of cultivated blueberries (berries grown to eat) has 9,019 antioxidants. Lowbush (or wild) blueberries have 13,427 total antioxidants per cup.

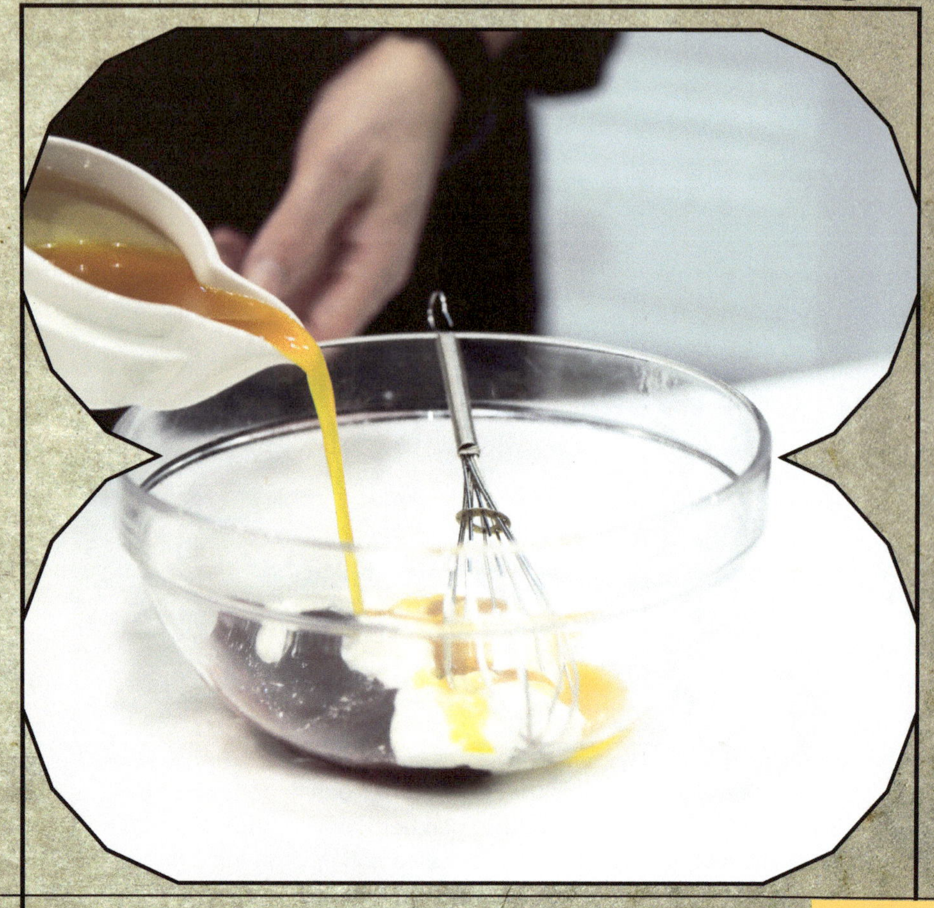

SAUCES AND SUBSTITUTES

HOW TO USE APPLESAUCE INSTEAD OF *oil*

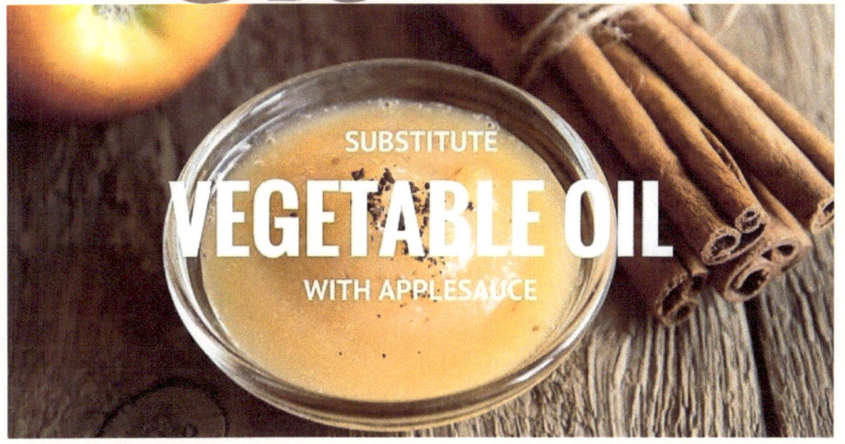

Applesauce can be used as a substitute for oil in baking recipes.

1. To replace oil with applesauce, use equal parts of applesauce in place of the oil. For example, if a recipe calls for 1/2 cup of oil, use 1/2 cup of applesauce instead.

2. Keep in mind that using applesauce in place of oil may result in a slightly different texture or flavor in the finished product, but it is a healthier option that can also add some natural sweetness to the recipe.

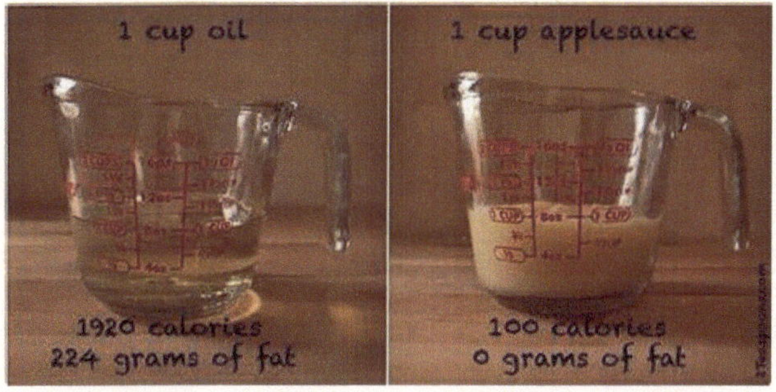

5 Minute Gratitude Journal

__/__/___

S M T W TH F S

Breath before writing

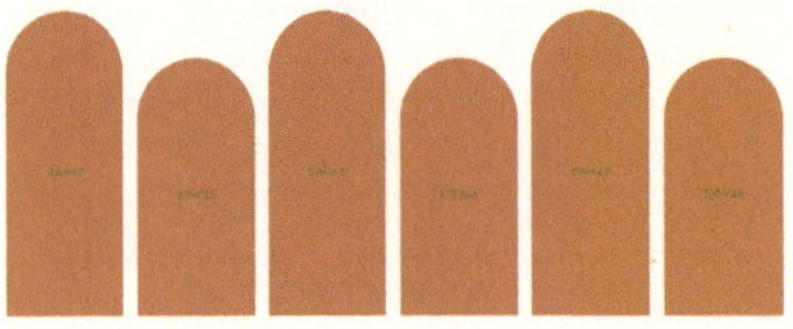

Things you're grateful today

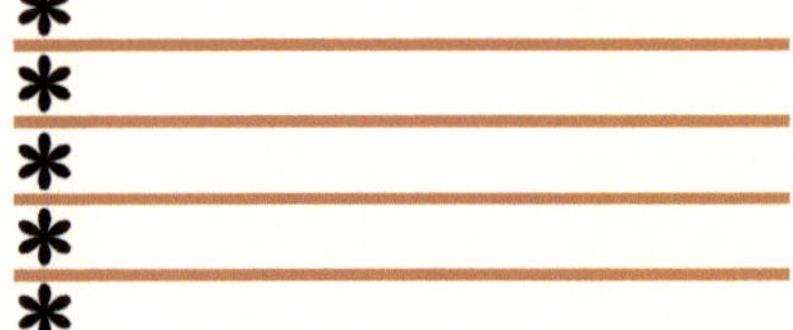

3 best thing about today

Today's Highlight

Describe today in a drawing

Things that you learned

Today's Affirmation

Today I'm grateful for...

HOW TO USE APPLESAUCE INSTEAD OF eggs

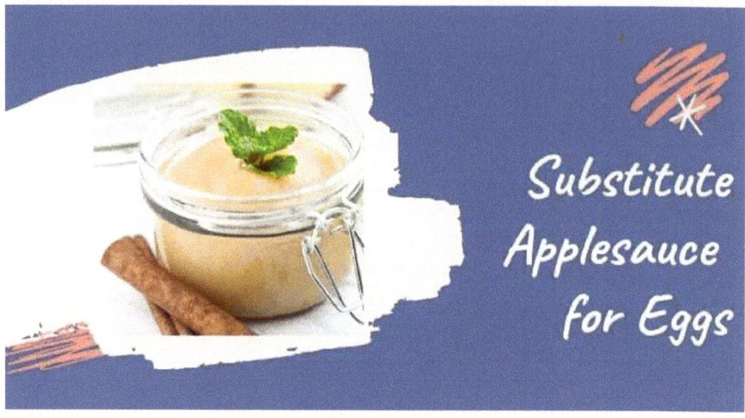

1. Applesauce can be a great substitute for eggs in baking recipes, especially for those who follow a vegan or egg-free diet.

2. To replace one egg, simply use 1/4 cup of applesauce.

3. This works best in recipes that call for one or two eggs.

Applesauce can add moisture and a slightly fruity flavor to baked goods, so it is best used in recipes where this flavor profile is desirable.

Keep in mind that using applesauce instead of eggs may result in slightly denser baked goods, but it is still a great option for those who want to avoid eggs.

1 cup applesauce

1 egg

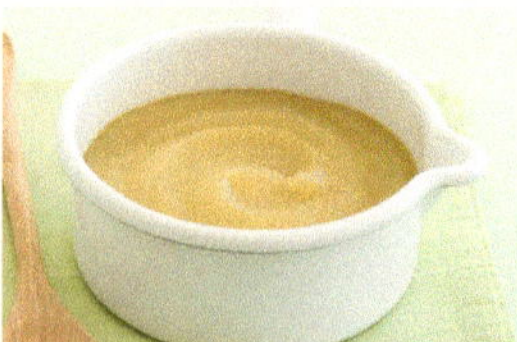

=

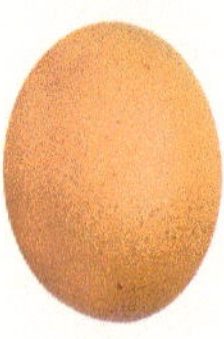

APPLESAUCE BARBQUE RECIPE

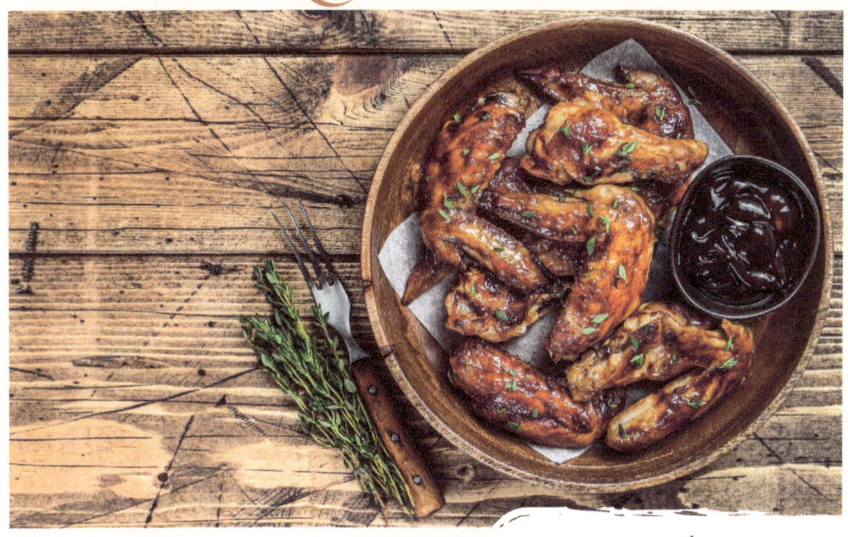

- 1 cup of applesauce
- 1/2 cup of ketchup
- 1/4 cup of brown sugar
- 1 tablespoon of apple cider vinegar
- salt
- pepper
- garlic powder
- onion powder

1. Mix 1 cup of applesauce, 1/2 cup of ketchup, 1/4 cup of brown sugar, and 1 tablespoon of apple cider vinegar in a bowl.

2. Add salt, pepper, garlic powder, and onion powder to taste.

3. Use the sauce to baste your meat while grilling or baking.

Enjoy!

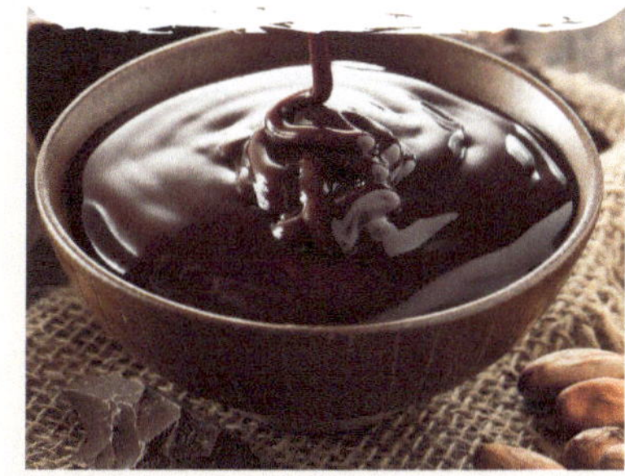

APPLESAUCE STEAKSAUCE

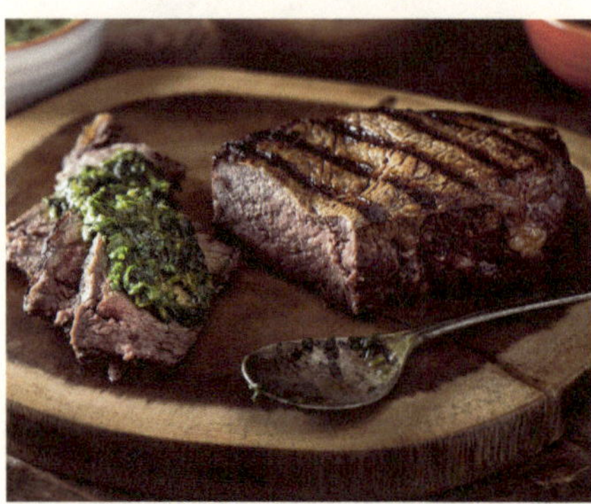

- 1 cup unsweetened applesauce
- 1/4 cup brown sugar
- 1/4 cup ketchup
- 1/4 cup apple cider vinegar
- 2 tablespoons Worcestershire sauce
- 1/2 teaspoon garlic powder
- 1/2 teaspoon onion powder
- Salt and pepper to taste

1 In a medium saucepan, combine all ingredients and stir until well blended.

2 Bring to a boil over medium heat, stirring occasionally

3 Reduce heat to low and simmer for 15-20 minutes, or until the sauce has thickened to your desired consistency.

4 Remove from heat and let cool before serving.

5 Enjoy your delicious homemade applesauce steak sauce with your favorite steak or other grilled meats.

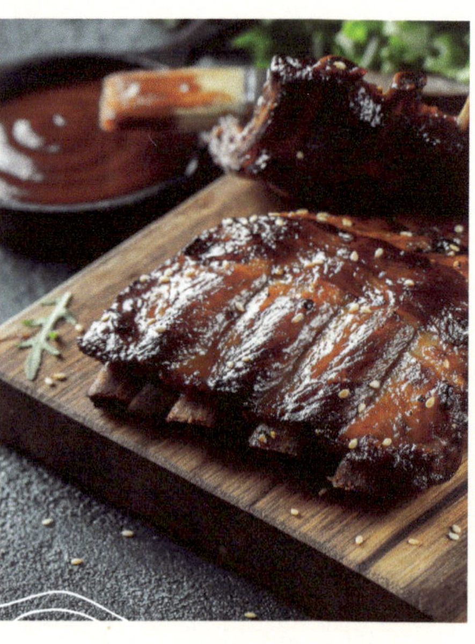

Today I'm grateful for...

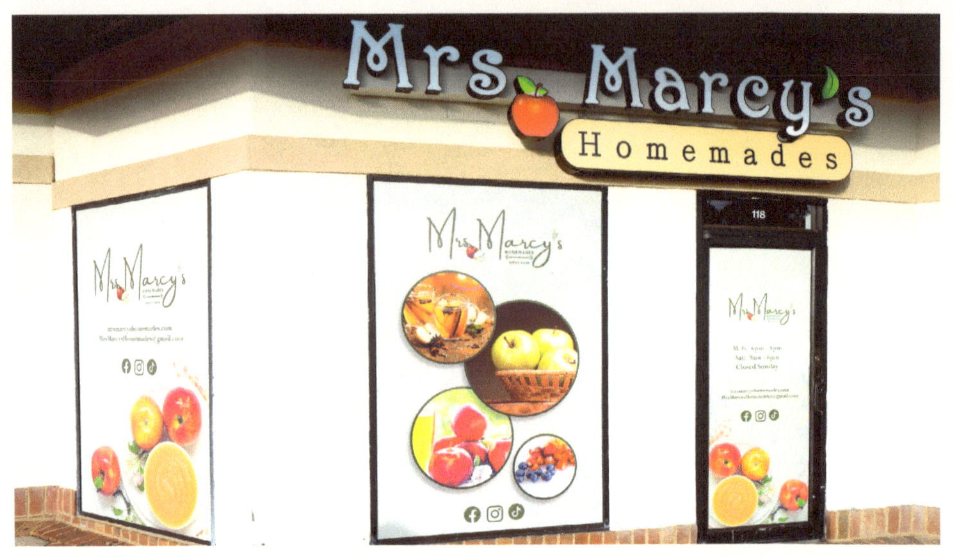

Mrs. Marcy's Homemades, LLC

['misiz, 'misəs] [mahr-sees] [ˌhō(m)'māds]

Founded 2020
Location: Richmond, Virginia
1st Black Woman-Owned Applesauce Manufacturer
SWAM Certified
Trademarked 2023

OUR PARTNERS

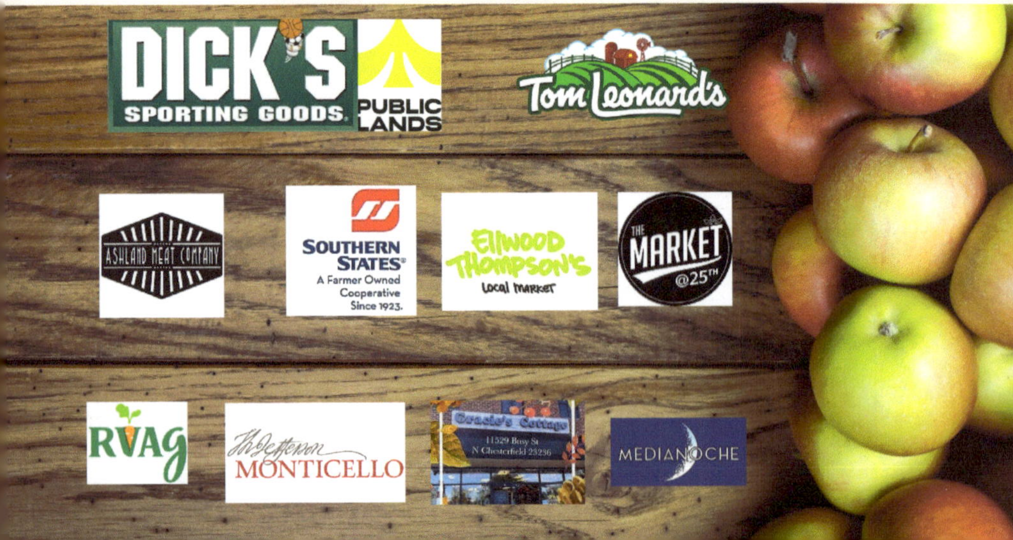

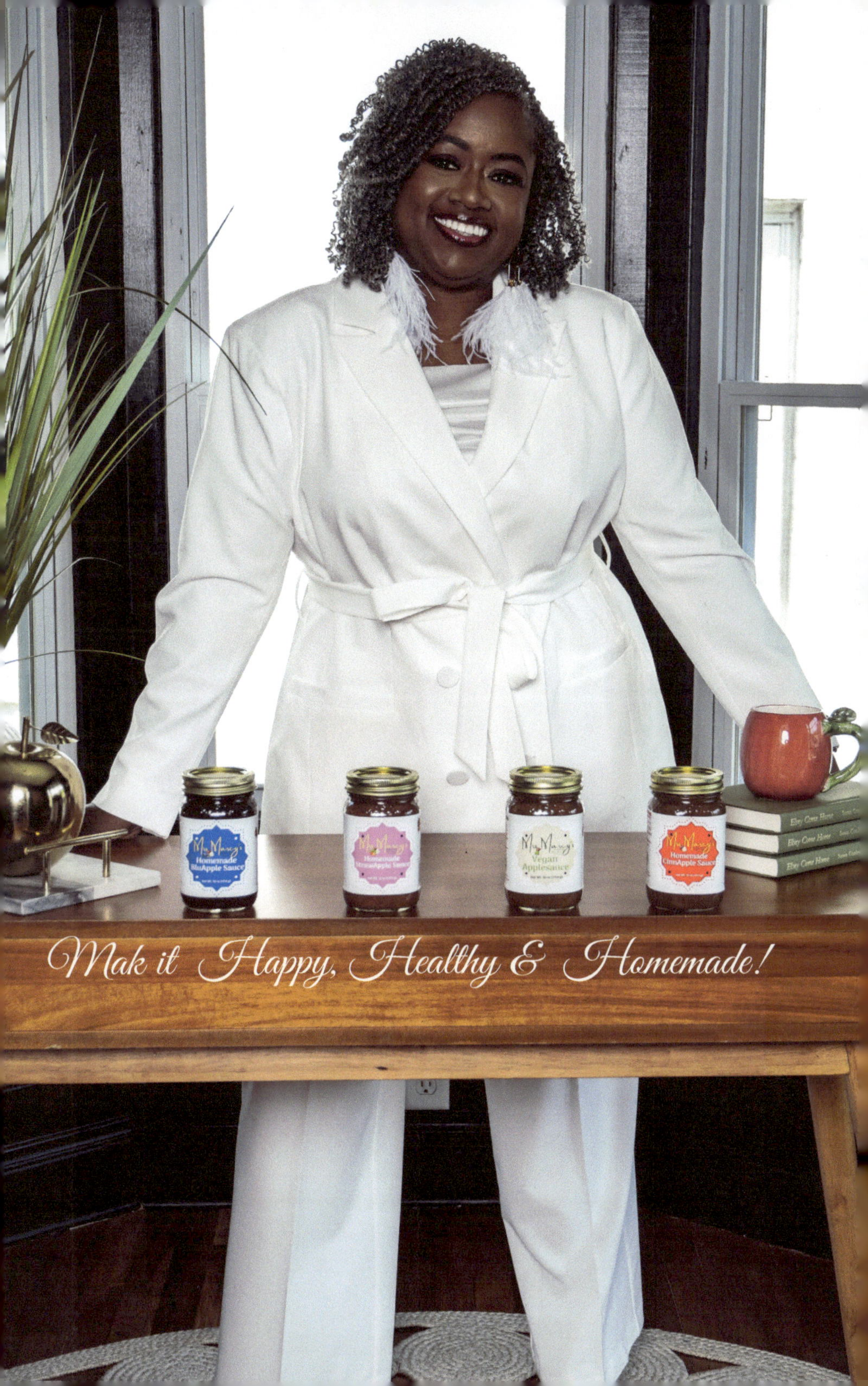
My Marcy's
Homemade
BluApple Sauce

My Marcy's
Homemade
StrawApple Sauce

My Marcy's
Vegan
Applesauce

My Marcy's
Homemade
CinnApple Sauce

Mak it Happy, Healthy & Homemade!

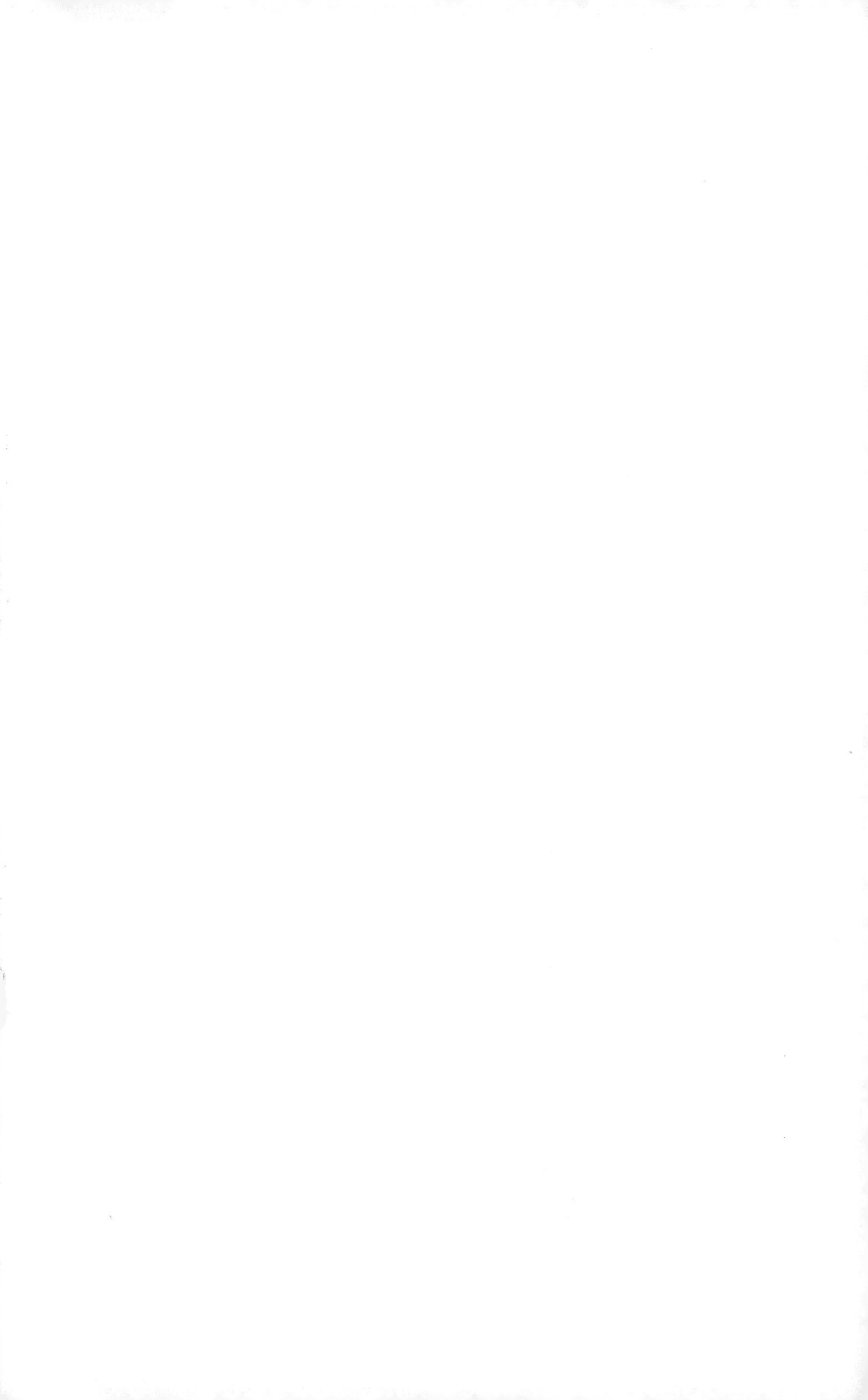

9 798853 842533